Dare...
to Try Bondage

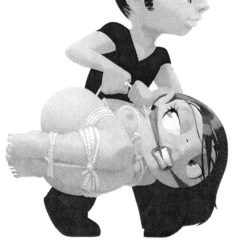

Other titles in the Positively Sexual series

Dare… to Have Anal Sex by Coralie Trinh Thi

Dare… to Have Sex Everywhere but in Bed by Marc Dannam

Dare… to Make Love with 2, 3, 4…or More by Marc Dannam

Dare… to Try Bisexuality by Pierre des Esseintes

Dare… to Try Bondage by Axterdam

Dare… to Try Kama Sutra by Marc Dannam and Axterdam

AXTERDAM

Dare...

to Try Bondage

Hunter House

Osez… le bondage © La Musardine, France, 2005
Translation © 2009 Hunter House Publishers, Alameda, CA

Hunter House Inc., Publishers
PO Box 2914
Alameda CA 94501-0914

Library of Congress Cataloging-in-Publication Data
Axterdam.
[Osez le bondage English]
Dare to try bondage / Axterdam. — 1st ed.
p. cm. — (Positively sexual series)
Includes bibliographical references and index.
ISBN 978-0-89793-514-2 (pbk.)
1. Bondage (Sexual behavior)   2. Sexual dominance and submission.   I. Title.
HQ79.A98 2009
306.77'5—dc22   2009012542

Project Credits

Cover: Brian Dittmar Graphic Design	Editor: Alexandra Mummery
Cover Illustrator: Arthur de Pins	Publicity Associate: Sean Harvey
Book Production: John McKercher	Order Fulfillment: Washul Lakdhon
Copy Editor: Amy Bauman	Administrator: Theresa Nelson
Proofreader: John David Marion	Computer Support: Peter Eichelberger

Senior Marketing Associate: Reina Santana
Rights Coordinator: Candace Groskreutz
Customer Service Manager: Christina Sverdrup
Publisher: Kiran S. Rana

Printed and Bound by Bang Printing

Manufactured in the United States of America

9 8 7 6 5 4 3 2 1   First Edition   09 10 11 12 13

Contents

Note: Some books quoted in this work have English-language editions; our text is translated from the French original and may not match the exact wording of the published English text.

Foreword to the U.S. Edition

by Yvonne K. Fulbright, PhD

◉ ...the Series

Leave it to the superbly sensual French to make the exotic all the more erotic, enticing, and accessible with the most charming set of sex books ever released.

When I first saw the *Osez...* (Dare) series, I was instantly seduced by the playful, titillating covers of this set of more than twenty pocket books. Delightfully disarming, these works inspire one to take on all taboos, summoning lovers to unleash their sexual nature as never before. Talk about *ooo-là-là*—these books leave no doubt as to why the French are known the world over for being sexy. Whether it is their food, wine, fashion, or simply their sensual language, the French are credited and revered for encouraging eroticism.

...all of the necessary knowledge and skills for... one of the "extreme sports" of sex

◉ ...this Book

For years, French artist Axterdam has been delighting audiences with his "primal" art, graphically portraying the human body's eroticism in dance, relaxation, self-pleasuring, and mutual pleasure. To say his works are at times a little bit naughty is an understatement. Such is the flavor of his *Dare... to Try Bondage*, one of twenty-four works from the *Osez...* (Dare) series, translated into Portuguese, Spanish, Italian, and now English, for lovers to enjoy. *Dare... to Try Bondage* captures the soothing, easy ebb and flow of lovers engaged in the ritual of physically restraining one partner for the other's pleasure and their own.

Rooted in Japanese bondage practices, the work reads like an erotic freefall, with Axterdam serving as your safety net and trainer. With a heavy emphasis on sex communication and the rules of this erotic engagement, the author takes a safety-first approach in this crash course on the joys of bondage. Readers are provided with all of the necessary knowledge and skills for what is regarded as one of the "extreme sports" of sex.

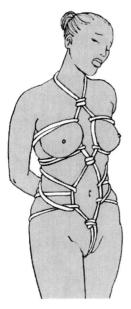

This succinct and complete training program reviews everything lovers need to know, providing detailed instruction on time-tested techniques and equipment. Axterdam also guides lovers in taking action outside of the bedroom, adding elements of fantasy and role-playing. Axterdam normalizes this often misunderstood behavior as he highlights the emotional pleasures to be had by the dominator and dominated. He advises readers on how to deal with sensory overload and how to safely come down from this super-charged erotic experience. And he does so with nothing short of the classiness for which French lovers have always been revered.

So check your gear and suit up. You're about to skydive into some of the most scintillating sex of your life.

— Yvonne K. Fulbright, PhD, MSEd
Professor of Human Sexuality, Argosy University
Coauthor, *Your Orgasmic Pregnancy*
Author of *The Hot Guide to Safer Sex* and *Touch Me There!*

Important Note

The material in this book is intended to provide a review of information regarding the practice of bondage for sensual and sexual pleasure. Every effort has been made to provide accurate and dependable information. We believe that the sensuality advice given in this book poses no risk to any healthy person. However, if you have any sexually transmitted diseases, we recommend consulting your doctor before using this book.

Therefore, the publisher, authors, and editors, as well as the professionals quoted in the book, cannot be held responsible for any error, omission, professional disagreement, or dated material, and are not liable for any damage, injury, or other adverse outcome of applying any of the information resources in this book. If you have questions concerning the application of the information described in this book, consult a qualified professional.

Warning!

Bondage can present real physical risks. These risks can be reduced if you follow the precautions and instructions described here. The author and the editor decline all responsibility for any eventualities or accidents that may result from attempting to practice situations described in this book.

Introduction

◎ The Confessions of an Accomplished
Bondage Artist (I swear!)

I am one of those people who is attracted to the submissive-dominant dynamic in erotic games and, more specifically, to bondage.

I have been practicing this art for many years. Initially, my bondage play involved binding myself. But then I discovered the pleasure of being restrained by others after I met a young woman named Aline, who had the gift of building sexual anticipation in a most delicious way.

Wanting to share my discovery with my friends, I began to organize bondage sessions and parties, adding my own personal touches. And my interest in bondage quickly went beyond simply interest or sensual pleasure. You see, I am a sketch artist and painter; soon, images of beauties stretched out submissively before me became my favorite subject. In a few years I had created hundreds of drawings of people in bondage, and I collected them all in a book published by La Musardine under the title *Carnets d'un obsédé* (An Obsessed Person's Notebook).

Thoughts for this book began to brew when a male friend became intrigued by the idea of bondage and began to ask lots of questions. Among other matters, he wanted to know:

- ☞ How do you tie the knots?
- ☞ What is it about this that excites you?
- ☞ How long can one stay tied-up?
- ☞ Where do you do it?

My female friends, on the other hand, never ask such questions. They have already, for the most part, witnessed the act—or have been the subject, themselves—of my bondage sessions. That does not mean that they know how to tie the bonds themselves. In any case, attempting to answer these types of questions makes for a very long conversation, so, instead, I offer them to you here, "wrapped up, tied with a bow" in this well-illustrated little book.

◉ **Shibari and Bondage**   The art of bondage is part of the greater family of sadomasochistic (S&M) activities. Since "soft" S&M practices first appeared in the sex lives of Westerners, people have become fascinated with the inspired restraints and devices of the Japanese quasi-philosophical expression of the master/servant relationship. For advanced practitioners, bondage is a lifestyle and a beautiful expression of sexuality; it implies a true understanding between the two participants. Yet, even as a manifestation of obedience from the submissive to the master, the ritual of Shibari* has more to do with simulation and role-playing than with putting a partner in true danger. The point is not to effectively restrain a prisoner; instead,

* *Shibari* is a Japanese word that literally means "to tie," or "to bind." It is used in Japan to describe the artful use of twine to tie objects or packages. *Kinbaku* is the word for "bondage" and there is also *Kinbaku-bi* which means "beautiful bondage." The word *Shibari* came into common use in the West at some point in the 1990s to describe the bondage art of Kinbaku.

it is meant to build anticipation. The anticipation is exquisite "torture" (and, as such, most delicious)—and should be much more wonderful than the act itself.

HISTORY OF BONDS Since ancient times the Japanese have had a special affinity for knots. We find representations of knots and ropes on ancient pottery symbolizing the relationship between humanity and the world of the gods. Shibari, or the art of Japanese erotic bonds, finds its true origins in the course of the "Dark Ages," around 1450, during what was called the Sengoku period, and it has remained popular among Japanese sexual practices to the present day.

Originally, techniques for tying bonds were used by soldiers and adopted by the samurai for the purpose of immobilization and to torture prisoners of war. The techniques were also used to imprison and punish lawbreakers. Shibari can even be used as a method of capitol punishment, since the penal code allows for several types of public punishment, one of which is suspension, ultimately resulting in the death of the prisoner.

Later, Shibari transformed itself into a military ritual before becoming a type of quasi-artistic punishment around the Edo period (1600–1868). An actual code governed the practice of this art: Ropes had different colors according to the time of year so that the prisoner had an indication of the change of seasons. Through the centuries, the rules evolved further, thus permitting one to know the prisoner's profession and the type of crime he or she had committed as well as the social position of the victim. Artists made many works depicting these costumes and rituals. Many aspects of Japanese civilization, in fact, are built on ritual; for example, making flower bouquets, practicing martial arts, sewing a kimono, and drinking tea. These rituals both recall ancestral traditions and create an intrinsic aesthetic. This is certainly true of the theater and extends into the realm of the erotic. Kabuki theater, in fact, would often present scenes of torture with sexual undertones.

The art of binding knots almost disappeared from Japanese tradition with the Westernization of the country. Nevertheless, in the middle of the twentieth century, an artist, Ito Seiu (1882–1961), sensationalized Shibari. Thanks to his numerous prints and an illustrated work titled, *The Hell of Tortures*, he brought the art of binding knots to the common people. And in approximately 1950 the first Japanese erotic magazine featuring Shibari content appeared; it was called *Kitan Club*. Following this literary introduction, and throughout the 1960s, many specialized magazines appeared, and Shibari eroticism bloomed. Erotic movies were produced as well, the most notable being from the famous Nikkatsu studio. These productions featured the delectable and ravishing submissive, Naomi Tani, who was shown tied-up in *Wife to Be Sacrificed* and *Woman in a Box*.

These days, the Japanese still practice Shibari for relaxation, relieving the stress and tension that is associated with the social constraints of their lifestyle. "Bondage parties" can be found in Tokyo, organized by young Japanese in leather masks and a combination of latex. Chimuo Nureki, master *sensei* of the classical school, organizes bondage sessions for a handpicked audience of enthusiasts.

It is impossible to tell the story of the history of bondage in Japan without mentioning the revolution that took place in the 1990s. The end of the twentieth century saw the evolution of the woman's role in the Japanese erotic scene, and the Japanese dominatrix was born! Not only does the dominatrix take the role of "master," but she also demonstrates a deft ability to tie up her subjects! That the Japanese man can allow himself to be humiliated by a woman is in itself a small tsunami in the Japanese social order.

But do not think that Japan has exclusive rights to the use of rope. During the 1950s the United States experienced its golden age of erotic photography with the introduction of Betty Page, pin-up and fetish fashion starlet, and the appearance of magazines glorifying beautiful women in bondage. And finally, in Europe in the beginning of the new millennia, Shibari attracted artistic photographers, for whom bondage creates something akin to a sculpture or a new way to show physical architecture.

Bondage will, without a doubt, continue to be a developing and evolving sexual practice. Couples are always looking for new ways to spice up their sex lives. So, in many ways, this guide addresses itself specifically to them. Bondage is a practice adapted to the times in that it is "safe." The practice of bondage is essentially based on the consent of both partners. Unlike sex in the days of carefree sex with strangers, bondage is not aimed at achieving sexual penetration. Rubbing, stroking, imperceptible caresses, whispered words in the ear, gentle slapping or spanking, and a touch of the whip are all allowed!

The word *bondage* is a fourteenth-century Middle English word. Its root, *bond,* means, "to attach; to stick together; or to form a union, obligation, or agreement." This always reminds us of the moral contract that exists between the partners.

Ch 1. **Are You Ready?**

Maybe you have fantasized about the drawings of Gwendoline, or John Willie, or of "Druuna" by Serpieri. Perhaps you love the photos of Araki, of Gilles, of Berquet, and of Romain Slocombe. Or maybe you have always been haunted by the images of Bettie Page, the films of Masaru Konuma, or *The Story of O.* Maybe for months now your spirit has wandered, and you have fantasized about yourself as a poor student subject to the discipline of a stern professor. Or, quite the opposite, maybe you have fantasized about having your beloved at your feet, defenseless, hands tied....

Are you sinking into the dregs of sexually perverse obsession? Your psychiatrist would need only a few minutes to surmise that you are ready for the leap into the realm of sadomasochism! And if he has had only a glimpse of the thoughts of Ito Seiu—Japanese master of Shibari—he might add that you are taking the first steps on the way to experiencing bondage! So, like innumerable Japanese who have practiced this six-hundred-year-old art form, rope bondage intrigues you....

I suggest that in the beginning you keep it simple, take time to study the rules and guidelines, do lots of research, and move forward very gently toward ever more subtle delights.

◉ **Golden Rules** Bondage consists of strapping your partner's body in an erotic or aesthetic position. It falls into the category of freely practiced erotic games, but this absolutely does not mean that it is without danger.

WARNING: Bondage can be extremely dangerous if you don't know human anatomy and/or don't understand and follow the basic rules—rules that are just plain, good sense.

If you want to hold a bondage session, it is essential to know and respect the following safety rules. The submissive partner, called here the "submissive," must have perfect confidence that these rules will be obeyed.

RULES THAT CANNOT BE BROKEN Even an extreme practice like bondage, which many people may consider immoral, has a code, with rules and limits. The rules of bondage are absolutely fixed:

- ☞ Do not injure your partner's body, hurt his/her feelings, or demoralize him/her.
- ☞ Never leave a tied-up person alone.
- ☞ Never discuss details of bondage sessions or techniques with strangers; doing so can result in all kinds of horrors.

BASIC RULES OF SAFETY Here are three safety practices everyone must follow:

You must always have a pair of scissors close by that can be used to cut the ropes. This is protection for you and your partner in case there is a stubborn knot at the end of the session, or if at any time during the session your partner doesn't feel well, cries out in pain, or is otherwise uncomfortable.

*You absolutely must have a code word or signal—understandable even if you use a gag—that both you and your partner agree **in advance** signifies the need for immediate release.* This signal can be a special wink, a hand gesture, or another indication that can be seen, heard, or felt even when the body is completely immobilized. My suggestion: The partner that is to be bound holds a small object in his or her hand, which can be released if need be. Hearing this object land with a thud should signal immediate untying, even if you have to cut your partner free with the scissors. Begin by immediately removing your partner's gag so that he or she can tell you exactly what the problem is (i.e., the rope is pinching or it is too tight on a part of the body).

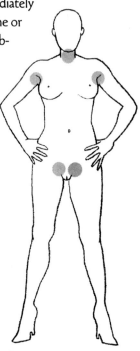

Never let a knot slip. As soon as a knot slips out of its original position, it becomes dangerous and may cause injury.

THE CARDINAL SAFETY RULE The figure to the right shows the three areas of the body that must never, under any circumstances, be restricted:

- the neck
- the groin
- the arm (at the armpit)

These are pathways for blood to flow to the heart!

The parts of the body that must never be restricted in your bondage play.

To avoid the effects of *blocked circulation* in the extremities, it is best to wrap a rope around sensitive areas—like wrists and ankles—a number of times. This spreads the binding over a greater surface area.

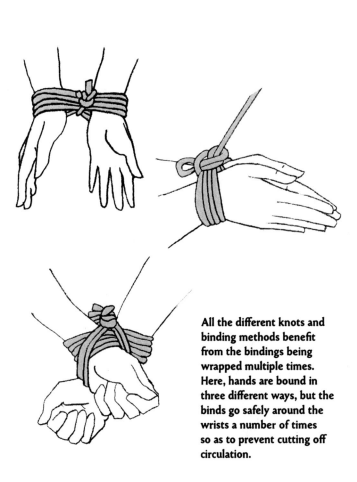

All the different knots and binding methods benefit from the bindings being wrapped multiple times. Here, hands are bound in three different ways, but the binds go safely around the wrists a number of times so as to prevent cutting off circulation.

Another cardinal rule: **Never keep a person restrained after they ask to be released**. Bondage is an erotic game that unfolds according to the wishes of a mutually consenting couple, in which both partners agree in advance to play nice so that everybody wins in the end.

The skin of your partner should be perfectly intact (i.e., there should be no cuts or other wounds) before the session begins. Even then, some materials are not recommended for binding your partner, because they carry a higher risk of injury. Among them are plastic chain, metal cable, rough rope, or plastic fiber (synthetic braid). For the same reason, you should not use handcuffs without padding!

If a prickling sensation, swelling, or discoloration develops around the binds, the knots must be undone immediately and the area massaged!

You should be aware of your partner's state of health. Are there concerns about circulation? Cardiopulmonary issues? A history of fainting or loss of consciousness? Know better than to bind the breasts of a woman who has had implants!

A FINAL WORD If you want to recreate your bonds from Japanese Shibari photos, be aware that the bodily dimensions of Asian people are different from those of many Western people. The average Asian waist is smaller and the buttocks are flatter, for example, which means that some configurations that work for a Japanese design will be impossible for Westerners.

And it is best to avoid elaborate suspensions, as seen in certain Japanese Shibari photos. These are spectacularly achieved on a set with a team of machinists, photographers, and experts. Sometimes it takes several assistants to hoist the model.

◉ **First Steps** You now know the safety essentials.

You should reconfirm one last time that your partner really wants to try this, that you are both in good health, that you are together on the plan, and that you have at least two full hours for the experience!

SUGGESTING BONDAGE TO YOUR PARTNER If you are a couple in the first few months of your relationship, you may find it very easy to suggest trying the sensuous practice of bondage. At this stage, when desire and admiration are over-whelming, it may be as easy as asking and all but a done deal. The best idea is to talk about it over the course of dinner: Bring up the subject and discuss it as a secret topic that will never be repeated to someone outside of the situation. Then set a date, or be spontaneous and get to it!

You may want to have everything prepared in advance—ropes, ambiance, setting, outfits—but if you don't want to wait, enjoy it now! Speak to your partner about what you want to do with his or her naked body, and she or he will likely not be able to resist your most convincing arguments.

If you are a more established couple, already comfortable in somewhat of a routine, try hiding your bondage materials close by the bed (under the mattress, behind the dresser, etc.) and wait for the moment. When the time seems right, reach for your secret treasure and suggest trying something new. Inspire your partner—he or she may take the initiative and run with it. Or, if you are the one receiving the suggestion, as soon as you try it, you may find you enjoy it; it amuses you. Try changing roles. Mix it up. You may find you grow as allies until—sud-denly—you brush up against the next level. Kisses mean some-thing more, a different emotion appears, the situation becomes erotic, and it is obvious that this is something that brings great pleasure that you can really share.

If it is your first foray into this pleasurable practice, go slowly! I strongly suggest you do not pounce on your partner with a rope and strap him or her down. That approach won't work unless you are with a professional model whom you have paid for this encounter or a young man recruited from a special site. At the very least make sure that your partner for the evening is someone who turns you on and in whom you sense a certain fearlessness.... Suggest that a little knot-tying session could be terribly erotic! The thing to look for is true interest and consent! You want to be sure about this.

Your partner may have to overcome the same apprehensions that you have or have had, so know how to answer the inevitable questions about everything under the sun. One must be persuasive and be able to quote texts, share attractive photos, and describe the sensuality of games played with anonymous others. (It is okay to talk about past experiences anonymously; no one will know the difference.) The key words here are *patience* and *courtesy*.

You may also have to address your partner's fears of being used. Tell your partner that true love does not seek to take advantage; assure her or him that no one will be ridiculed, that this does not lead to degradation, and that this practice is not to be confused with acts of depravity. While doing this, comfort your lover. Extol their beauty or explain that bondage is a way of glorifying the vision of their beauteous form. Convince your partner that they will be all the more beautiful for the way the knots magnify their features, especially when exposed by the designs of rope and the combination of knots on their skin, which you alone have learned to master.

Reading the above, one could get the impression that I am a silver-tongued salesman, a wordsmith, or a con artist. Not at all! To get what I want, I do not try to convince anyone. My playmates are "partners," or I would not even suggest the idea. Above all, I don't want to trick anyone. I want willing "prey."

The worst that can happen is you will be refused, either politely or furiously. But what's the harm of rejection in the life of a man or a woman? It is only a slap in the face to true love and the passing of an unpleasant moment.

In contrast, if it works, great rewards lie ahead!

◎ Pleasure

"Bondage with one or more partners offers many advantages: the real or simulated submission to the desires of another person, free from inhibitions, freedom from the guilt associated with a strict upbringing or shamed sexuality. One also enjoys orgasm free from responsibility for the sensations they feel: Bondage cures helplessness and frigidity. For a man, this submission alleviates his obligation to prove his virility. Consider that one who can break free from these bonds can regain a confidence in his or her self-esteem. It can also be reassuring to restrain a physically impressive partner: Some women feel a greater sense of security (after) putting a man in restraint."
— Brenda B. Love (translated from *Dictionnaire des fantasmes, perversions et pratiques de l'amour* [Dictionary of Fantasies, Perversions, and Love Practices])

There are many ways to experience pleasure while tied down with rope. They are all eminently cerebral.

THE PLEASURE OF THE DOMINATED Sometimes it is easier to lose control, to let go, and to approach orgasm more profoundly when you have totally submitted to the desires of someone else. One may reach an intense meditative state while immobilized and passive, like a solitary figure in the midst of a topsy-turvy world. At times it can be agreeable to stop making decisions, especially when, in your social or professional life, you assume great responsibilities and tend to be in charge.

Furthermore, by limiting certain senses (such as sight, with a blindfold, or speech, with a gag) or by disallowing the slightest gesture, one's spirit may be opened to a new world of receptivity to sensations.

In addition, feelings of shame, public ridicule, severe humiliation, or even terror can provoke real pleasure in certain types of partners with masochistic tendencies.

THE PLEASURE OF THE DOMINATOR How can one resist the temptation to dominate, to do whatever you want to do to someone else, to manipulate another's body and mental state, to take pleasure in the orgasm of the submissive partner? Bondage also offers aesthetic satisfaction, the pleasure of artistic creation, of making beauty, of demonstrating perfect confidence, and of being sensual.

◉ **The Ritual** A bondage session is a ritual. Each gesture is important; each thought counts.

ATTITUDE Bondage demands love, honesty, and respect. Its practice should procure pleasure for the submissive, for the master, and for any observers. It is in this light that I remind you of several precepts:

⇒ Practice immobilization only with your partner's consent.

⇒ Show respect for the ropes.

⇒ Appreciate the act of tying as much as its result.

⇒ Do not lose sight of the beauty of the subject.

One can compare the art of bondage with the tea ceremony. Both practices reveal a meditative thoughtfulness, a spiritual aesthetic tinted with perfumes, flavors, and sounds. It is a sacred moment. Prepare, think ahead, and set the scene: candles, soft or harsh light according to your tastes, props, music, heat turned to where you would set it in winter. Discover what brings you inner harmony....

If the décor is important, the dress code is, too. Once you have chosen a fantasy, dress the part. Dress up in costume and wear provocative underwear. Choose garments that "call out": silk, velour, leather.... Accessories are also important: a stylized mask, clean white ropes, a pearlesque probe (or clear dildo). Accentuate the room with dust, and perhaps you will find yourself in a medieval cave....

But at the same time be serious! Bondage takes place in an intense and dark ritual of severity; the situation is dire! Sensual, agreeable, but dire. To borrow the words of a friend raised in the Japanese culture, *"The Japanese don't kid around!"*

LANGUAGE The sexual masochist world revolves around the relationship between two people, where one is bound to the other's wishes. This type of relationship falls into the category of perversion in some people's estimation!

However, don't miss out on something intriguing because of another's viewpoint!

Start with some role-playing. There is an intrinsic dramatic composition to bondage that permits the use of a special vocabulary (heavy silences included!). Pleasure is shared in words, in the tone of voice, and in the subject. The master (or the mistress) must learn to command respect and give the correct orders. Whispering commands, not shouting them, is not for the first-timer. Basic rules include:

- Do not acknowledge a submissive; give clear, simple, and brief commands; alternate caresses and punishment.
- The submissive, for his or her part, should learn to obey and respond correctly. He or she should act with very little reserve and with respect but with just enough insolence to drive the domination through to the end of the night!

Each role player will find their own way....

RULE NUMBER ONE The submissive does not have a voice within this context; that's true. Still, you absolutely have to listen to their requests, for safety's sake. Your duty as master is to make sure you hear genuine complaints and act immediately.

DURATION Imagine that I spend

- 15 minutes binding my partner
- 8 minutes admiring the sight
- 5 minutes making a sketch or taking a tasteful picture
- 10 minutes caressing the beauty there
- 4 minutes untying

This means I have time for three poses in two hours, and this would be very pleasant indeed. But that is not the full essence of the experience; the essence is in hearing the pleasure of another...as it is in love, no?

On the other hand, if my tied-up friend desires to be plundered by three well-hung acquaintances while she is bound like a sausage, that could take some time. And in that case, one can't very well expect to attain more than a single pose within two hours! Too bad. But certainly she will be content.

CONSTRICTION As I want my partner to enjoy the experience with me, I am careful to manage her binds. For instance, I know that wrapping the ties around each member several times spreads out the forces of constriction, so I don't hesitate

---

WARNING! PAIN INCREASES THE LONGER YOU ARE TIED UP!

External signs of lesions are easy to spot. Look carefully at the color, the swelling, and the temperature of the skin around the binds:

- If the skin is cool and even-colored, all is OK.
- If the skin is warm, feels swollen, or has redness, take caution.

If you see any unexpected change to the skin, it is imperative you untie the knots and gently rub the tender area! Take action even before you see a change in color or evidence of swelling!

Further warning: Ten minutes seems to be the limit that an extremely uncomfortable position can be supported before irreversible damage occurs.

Note: Pay particular attention to how you tie bonds when working in low-light conditions, as you might find it more difficult to monitor any changes in skin tone.

to wrap and wrap. This may make my partner feel more at
ease, and my partner will be less likely to experience stifled circulation. Finally, to make sure that nothing is abrasive, I check
in with her about her comfort level.

PAIN   Must one cause or experience pain during a bondage
session?

"Aye," is my response!

The best response, actually, is that it depends on the
nature of the "ties" that exist between the two partners and
the agreement they have come to as a result of listening to
each other and trying to understand each other. If your partner
wants a little pain, why hesitate? If it is a question of sensitiv-
ity, try to specify a clear understanding. Furthermore, if your
playmate or lover has no taste for pain, why not try something
like silk scarves and loose knots or something more sugges-
tive. Because, obviously, it can hurt to be bound! Immobilization includes subtle and unintentional anguish; for example,
constriction can cause a loss of sensation in the extremities,
acrobatic positions can uncomfortably stretch the body, sensations of claustrophobia can result from being wrapped in rope.
During a suspension, there can be rope burns. It is all a matter
of training and understanding pain thresholds.

I knew a woman, a professional model, who could handle
it all: tight knots, flexed positions, piercing, gagging. I was
very impressed! What's more, her pleasure was proportional
to her expression of fear preceding the session and the pain
felt during it. She told me that since she went to pose for one
particular master, she passed through strange states—longing
for agony and restraints, wanting to do it for the money or out
of fear, aching for the stark reality of being stretched open or

immobilized. Blindfolded and vulnerable to the master's slightest whim, she felt an irresistible urge to find rock bottom! She didn't wish for it really, but the fantasy sometimes became so real that she would find herself shuddering on the verge of orgasm.

Ch 2. Supplies and Basic Techniques

There are a number of basic supplies you should purchase and techniques you should become familiar with before you start your explorations.

◉ **Ropes** A rope deserves respect from the submissive, the master, and its owner! It is the most intimate intermediary between the two actors. As such, it must be kept clean and in good order. It will be used to make designs on my darling's flesh and on her body. Personally, I prefer to use an all-cotton rope. I find this to be the most agreeable to

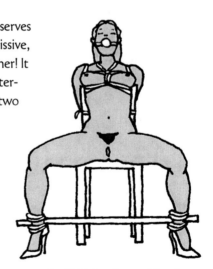

Blindfolded and immobilized, the submissive is vulnerable to the master's desires.

the touch—solid, pliable, and gentle when rubbing the skin. It is, however, difficult to find, expensive, and sometimes challenging to untie.

In general, next to cotton, everyone agrees on one type of material: the polyurethane rope. Made of nylon, it is pure synthetic; after several washings, it becomes soft and very agreeable to use. It is easy to find in hobby stores, sewing supply stores, outdoor equipment stores, or hardware stores. Nonabrasive, available in different colors (black or white works well), this rope allows for twisting into curls and making elaborate knots, and yet remains easy to untie.

I do not recommend any other types of rope! Some purists insist on hemp rope (fine woven), but it pricks, burns the skin, and is impossible to untie.

THE IDEAL ROPE The ideal rope has the following aspects:

- ⌐ diameter: ⅓ to ½ inch
- ⌐ material: cotton or polyurethane
- ⌐ length: 16 feet for binding just the limbs and between 40 and 50 feet for a full bondage; plus ends of 8 to 12 inches for decorative/finished tips
- ⌐ it is washed regularly
- ⌐ it can easily be cut with a scissors; the ends can be burned with a lighter
- ⌐ it can be rolled up or hung from something

◉ **Knots** To start with, a good simple shoelace knot will suffice. And if you have difficulty untying it, double the knot, but leave the loops in the knot to better define it. The first order of business for these knots is that they don't slip and don't constrict.

When you wish to experiment artistically, tie a flat knot (square), or what's called a security knot. (The security knot is less pretty, but, as indicated by its name, it is secure.) After these, you may learn to tie a double-8 knot, a grapnel knot, a cat's ear, etc. I will show each of these to you in this book (see below), but first, here are some pointers and rules.

To achieve a classic bondage pose, the knots must be tight, economical, strong, and beautiful! It is no small task. Practice finding the middle of the rope quickly; you can save time by making a small mark on the rope. One last thing: A rope that pulls across the skin leaves a burn! For me, it is very important not to mark my partners, especially when liberating them....

A good knot should

⇌ hold
⇌ be tight
⇌ be simple
⇌ be easy to untie

THE FLAT KNOT Advantages of the flat knot include that it:

⇌ is economical/efficient
⇌ does not slip
⇌ is aesthetically pleasing
⇌ is easy to tie
⇌ is easy to untie

≋ **Method:** Tie a shoe knot and then continue as if doubling the knot. But this time, loop the top string around and through toward its tail, not inverted as the first shoe knot. Pull tight.

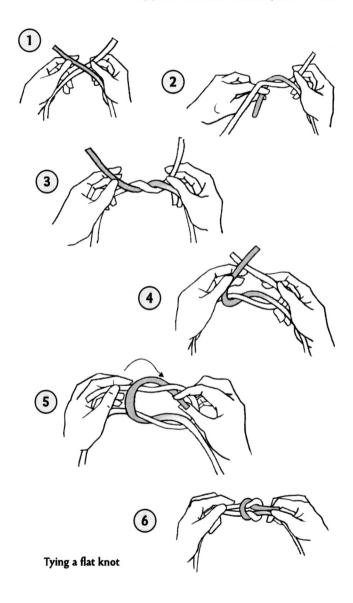

Tying a flat knot

THE SECURITY KNOT The advantages of the security knot include that it

- is quick
- is simple
- does not slip
- springs open instantly

The disadvantage is that it holds rather than tightens.

≈ **Method:** Make a shoe knot, but instead of passing the loose end through, pull a loop through and leave the loose end in the knot. Pull tight with the loop.

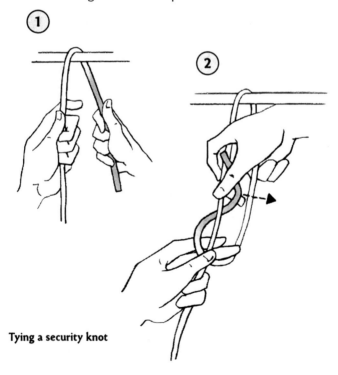

Tying a security knot

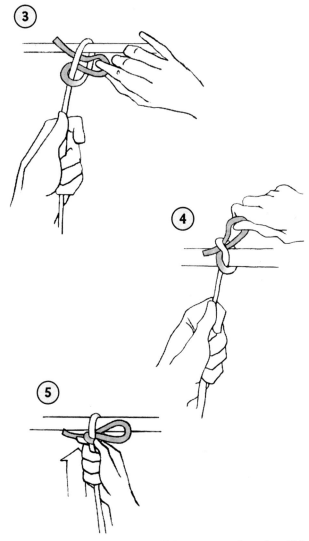

Tying a security knot (cont'd.)

THE DOUBLE-8 This knot is used to attach a partner to a
cross-brace bar, with all the security necessary for a suspension
or the hanging of a limb.

≈ *Method:* Loop one end of the rope. Wrap it twice around
the bar. Pass the loop around the outside of the sleeve and
back through it. Pull tight; adjust for looks.

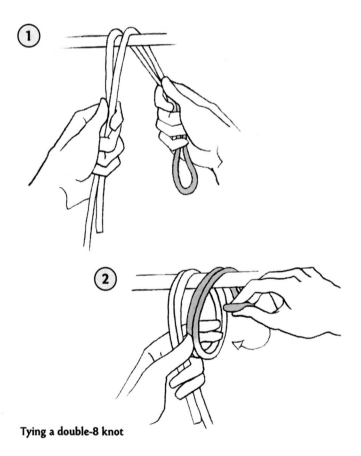

Tying a double-8 knot

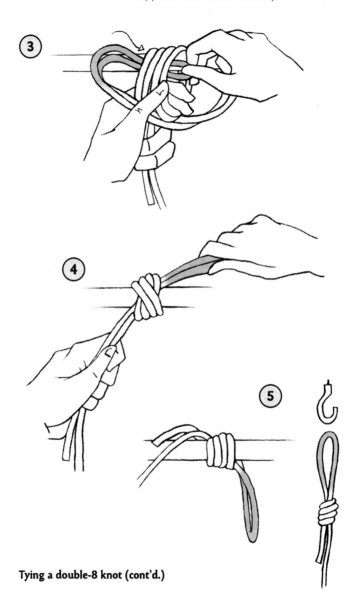

Tying a double-8 knot (cont'd.)

≈ *Tying the hands together behind (the back), crossed*
Finish by making a knot with the loop.

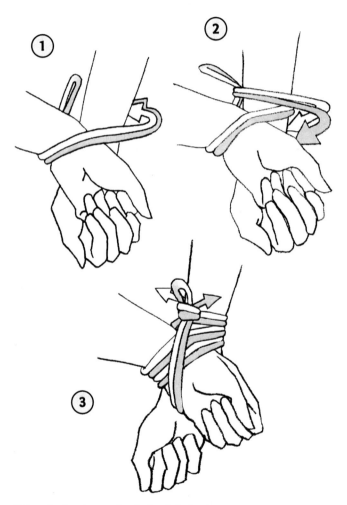

Tying the hands together behind the back

≋ Tying the hands together in front, parallel

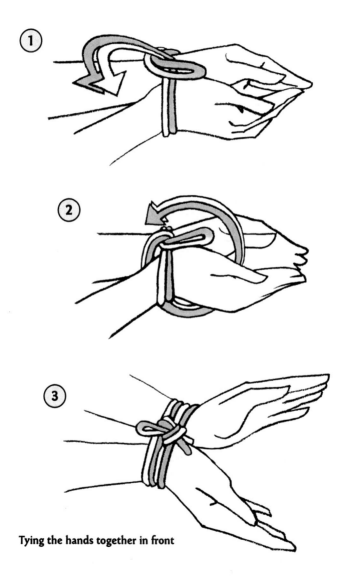

Tying the hands together in front

≋ *Tying the feet together in parallel*

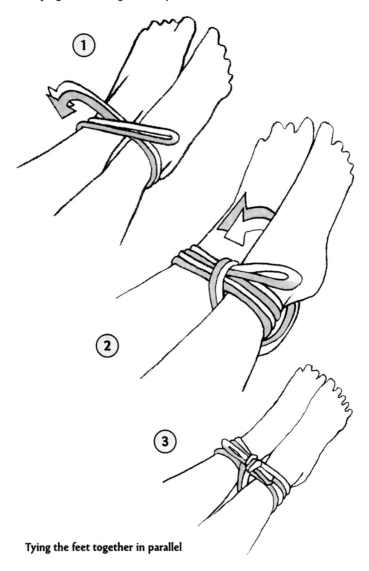

Tying the feet together in parallel

≋ *Tying the feet together crossed*

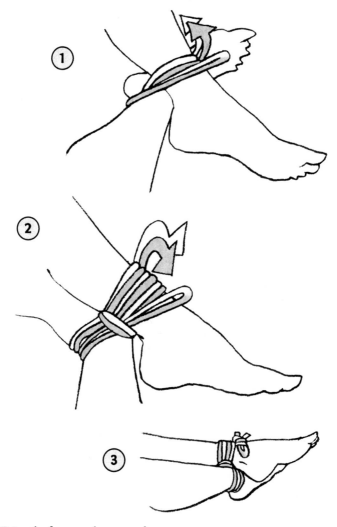

Tying the feet together crossed

◉ **Accessories** Tradition dictates that true Shibari is practiced entirely with ropes. Today, there is nothing that says you
can't use other, less conventional, materials.

Let's go over some of the more common nonrope materials: handcuffs, scarves, tape, pinchers, plastic wrap, the rack.

Handcuffs represent a strong symbol in the masochist domain.
Some people love them. I don't care for them. They hurt, they
don't hold to anything, and when you lose the key.... All that
said, the symbolism of handcuffs remains potent.

Scarves, stockings, panties, slips... these I adore! Whether
thin, thick, silk, cotton, solid or patterned, this is stuff of the
highest erotic value! The smells, the tears in the fabric, intimacy, everything is there for the fantasy. These accessories
allow, when used gently, using twists and tangles, the best
suspensions, and the prettiest immobilizations.

Tape also allows for elaborate harnessing! When you use
strong, wide tape, you can do wonderful things. But be careful
of the pulling! Loose hairs will be stripped off! This can be very
painful (although some people adore it).

Clothespins or other pinchers are obligatory for real maso-
chists. Think of replacing the brutish (but effective) clothespins with two chopsticks, fixed with rubber bands to pinch
the nipple. The result can be very pleasing to view.

Plastic wrap (film), which is normally used for food, can create
interesting effects for photos. The sensation of being squeezed
and stuffed while completely on display is extremely arousing
to many maso-exhibitionists. Beware, however: Wrapping the
head is absolutely prohibited: Breathing is vital!

Bungee/elastic cords, which can serve to replace rope, are like being caught by a spider. Pinching, pulling, and biting into the skin, elastic cords are definitely only meant for true "martyrs."

Ch **3.** The Session

You are well aware of the rules of safety that must always be respected. You have good supplies. You have practiced the skills. Your lover is into it.... It is time to begin!

To help you concentrate and to create a sense of touch between you, nothing is better than a gentle massage. This also gives your partner time to warm up, handle the ropes, and just get comfortable. Only then do I start to wrap our gift. Prettily tied! Nicely decorated. I try to have something in mind—a plan of action—before I begin. This allows me to free my submissive easily, if need be, by simply reversing my steps.

I think which limbs will be immobilized the longest and adjust the tightness accordingly. Those that will be bound

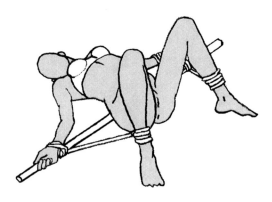

the longest, I don't tie as tightly. Then I finish with the tighter knots: for suspensions, arching and extension, the last body part touching the floor. (One can use cushions here and there shamelessly!)

Most of the time I start with the extremities, the hands and feet, and work my way to the center. An exception to this is a figure called the diamond; for this one I start as indicated on the following page.

Notice that the tying techniques are simple and quickly executed. In the field of bondage, I remain an eternal student, for I am always learning bits and pieces with every meeting and every practice—in this way it is a little like Buddhist or Taoist philosophy. These techniques are at once universal and unique. Take inspiration, copy them—and then find your own way!

Rules of Art; Rules of Gold The rules of bondage have already been set forth. Most of them are rules relating to safety. Yet there are other rules to learn, so long as they are not contradictory. Bondage has both aesthetic and erotic rewards. It is not enough to wrap someone in rope; you also want to transform your partner's body into a work of art.

- Respect symmetry.
- Devote yourself to the tension of the ropes.
- Avoid overlapping or twisting the rope.
- Respect balance in general.
- Let your work be guided by the elegance of the figure.

"The practice of bondage can be anywhere from simple to complicated. So, I'll make it simple, at the end of this draining afternoon [...] Nicole hasn't asked for the moon and is content to offer me her two arms. I have tied them to her back, in the imperial style. Other than the two lines of dark black that compress the melons, I have added a supplementary that connects to the hips and digs into her skin a little. They are tied to each other, for the purpose of limiting her movement, with a fourth that begins at the height of the navel and runs to the two superiors between her breasts and ends in a loop that is passed around her neck. It doesn't look like it, to see me do it, but this demands several weeks of apprenticeship...."

— Phiippe Djian (translated from *Vers chez les blancs* [Lines of White])

◉ Mune Nawa (Tying the Breasts)

≈ *Method:* Find the middle of the rope. Wrap the doubled-up line around the bust below the breasts and make a second round (passing through the loop). Send the loose ends over the shoulder and under the lines up front. Return over the other shoulder. Run the

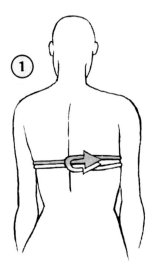

ends through the loop, under the lines that run around the
bust, and twice around the top of the breasts. Finish with a
pretty knot, such as a safety knot.

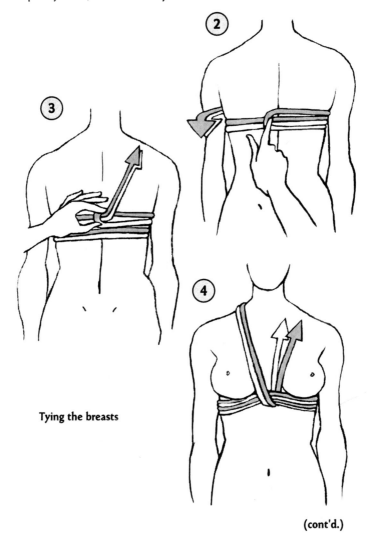

Tying the breasts

(cont'd.)

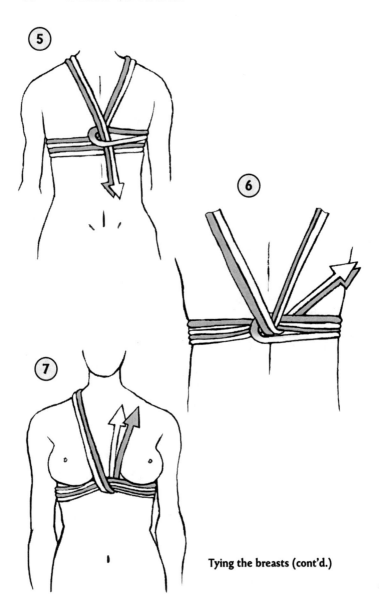

Tying the breasts (cont'd.)

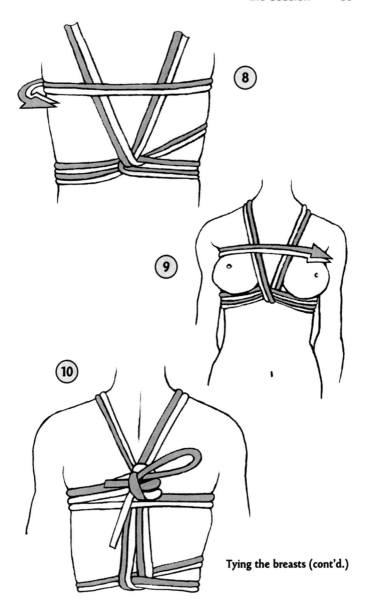

Tying the breasts (cont'd.)

◉ The Kikkou (Tortoise) Diamond

≈ *Method:* Hold the rope in the middle
and make a knot. Add a second knot
that leaves enough room from the
first knot to slip the rope over the
head. Place the head through
the split lines between the
two knots and make a knot
approximately every
8 inches as you drop
the rope down the
body. Bring the rope
up the back; pass the
loose ends through
the first loop and send
them around each side
(toward the front).

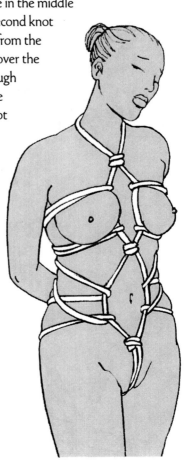

Tying the kikkou diamond

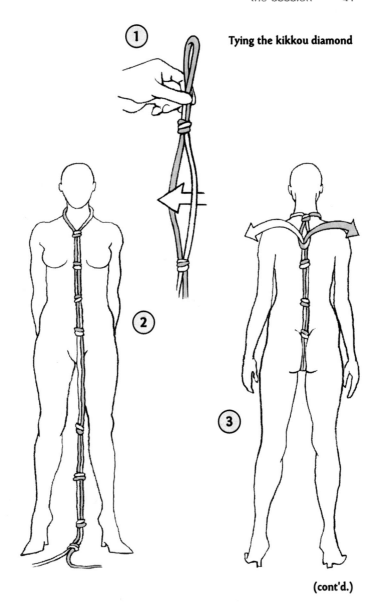

(cont'd.)

Insert each end in the split lines to lace the back of the torso, repeating about seven times. Finish there with the last pretty knot.

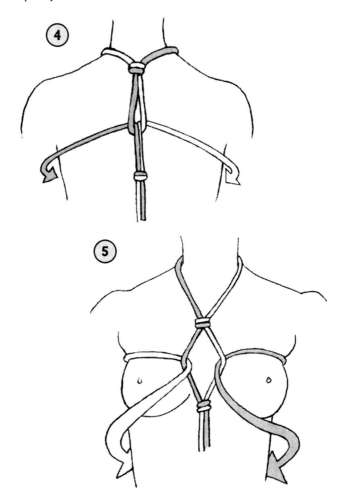

Tying the kikkou diamond (cont'd.)

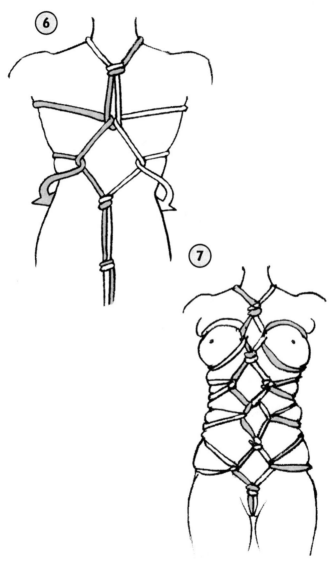

Tying the kikkou diamond (cont'd.)

≋ *Variation 1:* If your rope is long enough (50 feet minimum), continue tying all the way to the feet (see the figure below): The sensation is impressive!

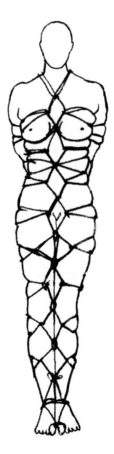

With this first variation, continue tying to the feet. It calls for more rope but is impressive.

≈ **Variation 2:** With a second rope (of equal or smaller diameter), bind the legs independently, as indicated in the sketches below. This one is guaranteed to be sensational!

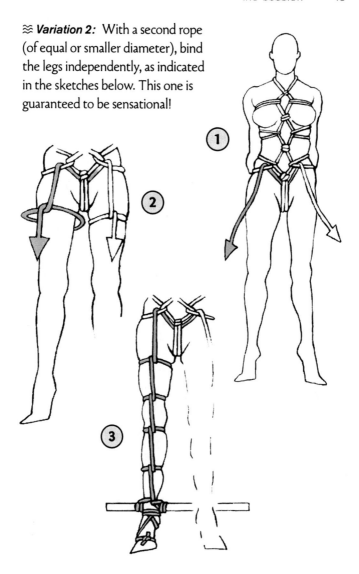

Tying the kikkou diamond, variation 2

"I am mad with excitement! A true beast! She has driven me mad! This girl is reserved, but I finally have her at the end of my rope. I started with a kikkou diamond tied with charm and softness; she is unaware that I have her hair tied also: That was not hard to accomplish with her tied up as she is! Still she tries to escape me! Now it is my turn to shake her little ass!"

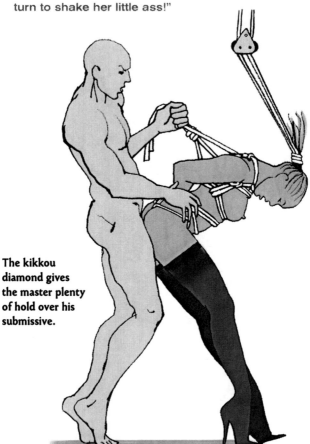

The kikkou diamond gives the master plenty of hold over his submissive.

◎ Ashitote Musubi (Hands and Feet Tied)

≈ *Method:* Hold the rope in the middle. Starting with the middle, wrap the ankles. Make a loop around the first loop. Wrap over the ankle ropes and then run the loose ends under the feet.

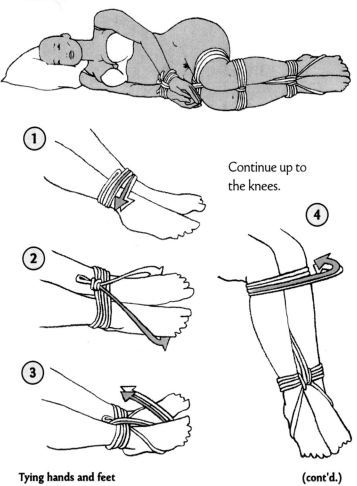

Continue up to the knees.

Tying hands and feet   **(cont'd.)**

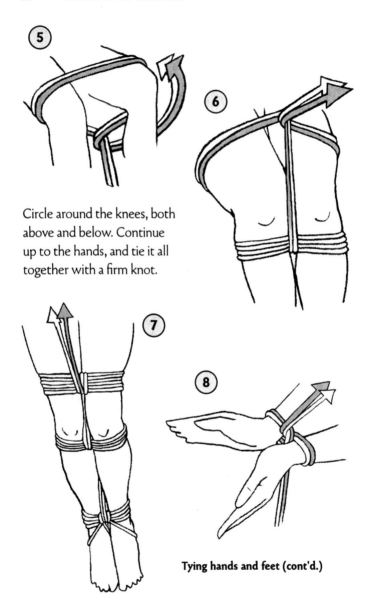

Circle around the knees, both above and below. Continue up to the hands, and tie it all together with a firm knot.

Tying hands and feet (cont'd.)

"I found myself abandoned for a while in this position. I finally relaxed. Closing my eyes, I thought I heard someone coming close: It was a man, and his scent was Asian. No! Indian! It was an exotic man...ohh! He put his hands on me, touching me. How softly, how apt! The feeling was incredible... I was being treated to an Ayurvedic massage. What luck! Thank you, my love!"

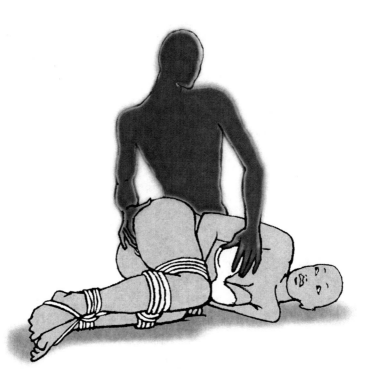

The master caresses his submissive, who is bound hand and foot.

◉ Gyaku-Ebi (Inverted Prawn)

≈ *Method:* Fold the rope in its middle; wrap around the ankles.

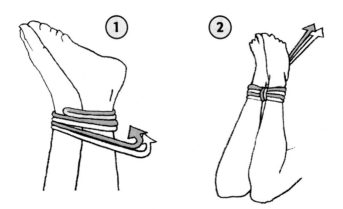

Wrap a second rope around the ankle ropes and continue toward the waist. Wrap around the waist; pull to bring ankles toward the waist. If you need to, make a knot to hold the tension. Wrap the hands; make a knot there also.

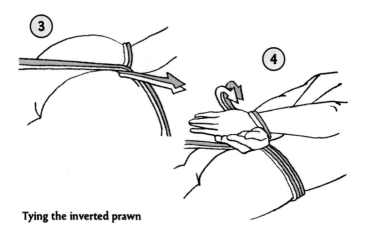

Tying the inverted prawn

Send the loose ends back around the "x" at the ankles; pull
and knot.

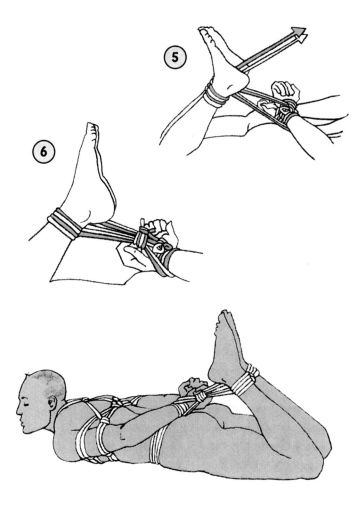

Tying the inverted prawn (cont'd.)

"This time the roles are reversed! The man has let himself be caught...how delicious. I waited for the right time, and now look what I've got. Lovemaking from this position is not so comfy; he must make an effort. I will take my delight from his pretty mouth! I think I'll have my pleasure where I please!... Do it, baby. Lick me, swallow me, and bury your nose right in it. Let your tongue caress me...."

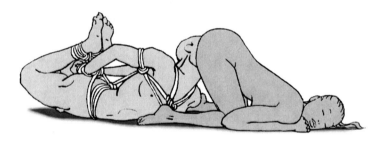

The pleasures that can be given to—and taken from—a partner in bondage are many!

◉ Kaikyaku Kani (Crab with Legs Spread Open)

≋ *Method:* Seat the submissive in the crab position (see image to the right). Tie the ankle and wrist together. Pass the loose ends underneath and through; wrap several times. Direct the rope toward the knee.

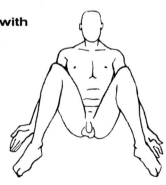

Submissive seated in crab position

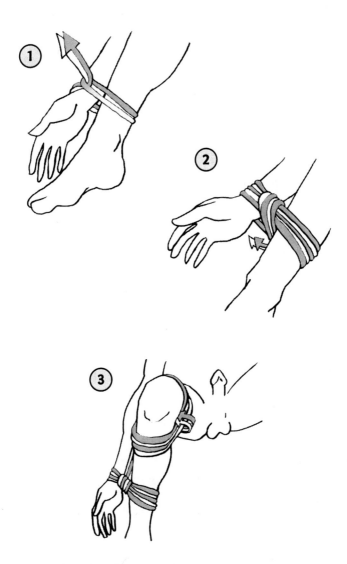

Tying the crab with legs spread open   **(cont'd.)**

Tie the rope beneath the knee. With another rope, repeat the tying steps presented above on the other ankle/wrist/knee. Finish by crossing ropes in front of torso and wrapping them around to the back of the torso. Make a knot in the back.

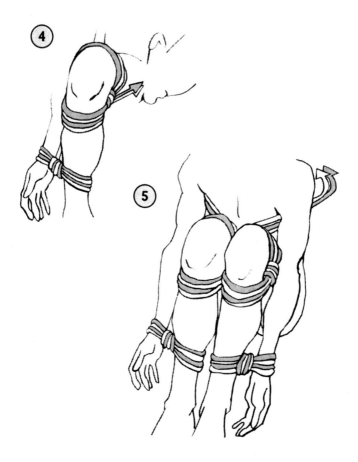

Tying the crab with legs spread open (cont'd.)

"I'm astonished you don't prefer this pose as a
rule. Poor little thing! Oh, I'll just put my hand on
your magnificent precious jewels...hiding in this
prison of legs and ropes. Oh, that must hurt! If
only you could get off...and with my skilled hands
I can help, though it will be hard...with you all
tucked up in there like that. It must be awful!
Mmm, I'll bet that feels better!"

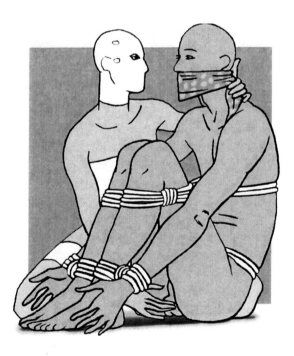

**Working your way through the web of bindings to
touch your partner's sensuous spots can bring many
moments of delightful anticipation for both of you.**

Johanna, a friend found on the scene, tells us of her forays into submission:

> "My husband was often away, and to kill time and forget my loneliness I would surf the Web for erotic sites. I love their stories. Most of all I love the stories about feminine submission—so much that I would stroke myself in front of the screen, fantasizing about what the writers described. One day, I happened onto a site where one of the published stories got me especially hot. There was an address for the author, and, one night, seeing he was online, I sent him an instant message.

> "In a few sentences he was able to sense my solitude as well as my desire to communicate and to procure my fantasies. He suggested some games, harmless at first, to feel out my submissiveness. Like putting a chain around my waist, handcuffs on my wrists, a gag.... To demonstrate that I would obey his orders, I was to send him pictures of myself from time to time.

> "He immersed me deeper and deeper into more severe submissions. Presently, for the duration of our conversations, I must wear two vibrators fixed to a chain strapped between my legs and around my waist. And that's padlocked. My ankles are tied to the legs of my chair; my wrists are trapped in cuffs that are tied to my neck by a chain. To write I have to lean forward and then rock back to see the screen. This motion grinds the two vibrators in my orifices constantly. My hands cannot reach my clit although I would

really like to. Then I could rub myself and appease the pain and the excitement...."

⊚ **Several Positions** Each goal and each stage can enhance the sensations that bondage brings.

    A CHAIR Madame is tied to the chair. Shall we play a game of balance? The chair, because Madame is strapped tightly to it, can be tipped (back). Madame can be the object of my most creative caresses....

"You have all the luck, Sabine... but now look at you! The market bounced well enough today... enough to save your skin! But you heard the news, too: Interest rates are up 0.7! And a 0.5 percent sales tax hike! It's going to be punishing for sure. There's nothing we can do there. But here, I make the rules. Come here and sit in the chair. Hike up your skirt! Thank you...."

Your partner, tied to a chair, presents all sorts of opportunities for fun.

A BED The bed is the perfect place for lovemaking. By combining the natural features of the bed with the ritual of bondage, you can discover a new world of pleasures. The ideal bed will obviously have bars; if not, what's the point? Iron headboards and footboards are getting harder to find, and a canopy bed...oh, to dream! But whether it is posts for tying to or a canopy to contain your most creative thoughts, a bed is ambience guaranteed.

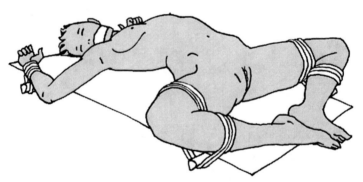

**Adding your bed to your bondage experience
can create the most interesting fantasies.**

"You are finally at Max and Martine's day spa to
the stars! You are being pampered...let go! We
will take care of your every need. Lie on this
table...open your arms and your legs. Don't be
shy. If I tie you up, it is so I can wax your bikini
line...and there! This scarf over your mouth will
keep you from getting too loud if you should want
to yell as the hairs are pulled from the hollow of
your most intimate crease...stretched open....
Martine is a master with her hands...."

A TREE A tree is a great prop for playing cowboys and Indians, or "lost in the jungle," or "tied to a tree naked in the forest." There are endless scenarios! What could be better? But a tree with privacy may be hard to find in the city. Instead, try using a garden gazebo to tie up your new conquests; it may present an interesting alternative.

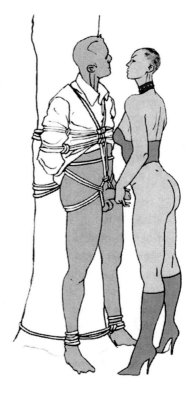

> "You love nature, you are drawn to the woods, and you will be drawn tight! I'm going to leave you here awhile, alone, with the animals. Maybe you will see a sly fox, a wild boar... or perhaps three lumberjacks who've come to penetrate this private grove. I'm sure they will not ignore such a beautiful caught dove.... Shouldn't there be some reward for letting you go?"

THE STAIRS A staircase or a ramp allows one to visualize as many complex poses as delights. Uncomfortable, serendipitous for restraints, the stairs are an ideal site for acrobatic bondage.

Do not forget to use other furnishings and various objects: posts, stools, bathtub, cage, corner, bars, beams, sling.... Each one of us can create our own smoking-hot scenario. Tied up naked in a bathtub like a mummy in a sarcophagus, suspended from a gymnast's rings, bent over a stool in the middle of the kitchen, shackled to a post like the victim of a meal promised to cannibals.... My God! You would be delicious tied up like that....

"Romantic Bond 14" is a bondage amateur who I found on the Internet. In April 2002 he told us of an evening he spent with a pretty girl and a smooth rope:

> "I have a fantastic connection with a woman who is close to me. With her, anything goes, and I have, thanks to her, realized a number of fantasies. Last night, when I went over to her place, she was waiting for me, on all fours and completely naked. In her teeth she held a thick rope that she had carefully run between her divine thighs. Submissively, she pitched forward, lying down, hands running the length of her body. I made her bend her legs at the knees and told her to spread wide. I ran the rope between her legs, over her belly and over her breasts, too. Once she was completely tied, she was even more exciting to me. With her legs spread open, she gave me a clear view of her moistening mound. Her breasts, almost crushed by the rope, made me want to slide my cock between them and squirm around for a long time. I pushed myself against her lips, and she had a good lick. When I slid a cushion under the small of her back, my

submissive arched a bit more, despite the ropes holding her in place.

"While she had her legs spread, her sex was tightly pinched by the ropes. And the hemp that passed over her button had worked its magic from the first deep strokes I took in and out of her. Usually, when close to cumming, she would dig her nails into my skin. There, tied up, she could not do it and saw fit to squeeze instead, so hard that it felt like her sex had a grip on me, so strong that we shouted out together when my juice gushed out into her loins."

Ch 4. The Sensations

What are the sensations felt by each partner? We have asked this question of a few friends in an attempt to establish some classification.

◉ For the Master or the Mistress

1. THE PLEASURE OF HAVING CONTROL "There's no way to hide it," says Sophie. "When I see a boy tied up, completely at my mercy and having to obey every one of my commands— 'Hold your hands out! Lift your arms! Stand over here!'—it makes me hot."

2. PLAYING "When she is completely restrained, she is nothing more than a pretty doll of flesh and of twine," admits Louis. "I take her, I give her back, I slide in-between her knots...."

3. GIVING PLEASURE "Immobile, my poor Loulou cannot defend herself when I take her sex in my mouth. Gagged, she can't even grumble! It is nothing more than great head," affirms Anna.

4. DEEPER PENETRATION "When she is well restrained, my darling is nothing more than an offering of sex. I slide myself into her depths; her immobility adds to my pleasure," says

Harvey—pardon, *Master* Harvey. "I see her look of surrender; I feel love."

5. TIGHTER SEX "Legs bound together by ropes, butt cheeks stuck together, my darling offers me her tiny ass. It seems firmer to me like that, and her little pussy is very, very tight," Louis says, adding that he almost has the impression of taking his submissive's virginity again.

6. ORGASM "That works for me!" responds a chorus of our friends.

7. FREEING "The end of the game is almost as pleasant as the first part," confirms Stephanie. "Untying each knot is a source of new pleasure."

8. MASSAGE (FONDLING) "Massage is an integral part of the pleasure," reports Louise at the end of a long session. "My master rubs each part of my body. He revives me after annihilating my senses for a while."

9. LOVE "Obviously," everyone says together.

10. KNOWING JUST WHERE TO GO (SELF-CONTROL)
"Bondage is also a school of responsibility," states John. "Each knot can affect the well-being—the outlook—of the submissive. One must be master of oneself."

11. DOMINANCE "Bondage is a 'soft' type of domination; it's the one I prefer," says Louise. "I have never wanted to hit a man or to scratch his face. By tying him down, I deprive him of the tiniest bit of power. And I reduce him to an object—an object of art!"

Jean-Claude Baboulin, bondage amateur, describes his practices in a book illustrated by Tonton Ficelle titled *Contraintes:*

"For twenty years or so, Charles and I have tied up young women and others not-so-young. In truth, he is the one who ties, and I content myself, generally, with assisting. In every sense of the term, I assist the 'master of bondage,' who sometimes needs help to realize this or that particularly complex figure, and I provide assistance for the spectacle, always fascinated and overcome with invention. I am also the photographer when a body composition or facial expression calls for it. Charles is much further along, obviously, in discovering a passion, which he has known [of] since adolescence. However, what I believe I have contributed is an introduction to certain 'subjects' of particular interest, as they are sincerely motivated and their passion has the same authenticity. From these introductions are sometimes born quasi-amorous relationships, based on an extremely erotic tension, total confidence in each other, and an understanding above and beyond words and gestures. Without a doubt, people like Laurence, Ghislaine, Brigitte...are included, as they have been able, thanks to Charles, to open themselves through total abandon to the 'banished part' of their sexuality. [...] One should understand, in the practice of bondage, the consent of the 'victim' is completely necessary but insufficient for a successful session. The tying of constraints creates the scene, and sometimes the suffering, requiring the advantages of passive acceptance: This demands engagement, the total abandon of the person in the position of submitting, man or woman—though with Charles it is almost always a lady. Sadomasochism (bondage being a variant of such) is the creation of a scene in the true sense of the term, a theater where our fears and anguishes are exposed, [as are] our boundaries, where the image we project of ourselves does not conform to social norms...."

◎ **For the Submissive (Man or Woman)** "I love pleasure," says Angela. "Bondage offers me a particular form: the pleasure of being an object of pleasure. What I like, what I adore, what makes me cum, is to be taken, isolated, handled, immobilized, possessed.... I like to become the pain and suffering of my master—I like to be punished, martyred.... Just as much, I adore the end of the session, when I am caressed, freed.... Knowing the sensation of loosening tension can be orgasmic. Bondage has allowed me to know my true fear, a pleasant vertigo, the anguish provoked by the loss of personal space, an adventure. And at the end of the story, I relish the reconnection with my liberator and love!"

Ch 5. **The Session May Be Over... but Not the Pleasure**

For those who appreciate marks left by the rope, the moment of "untying" is intense.

◉ **Untying** I can still feel the emotion in slowly and calmly letting the ropes slide over my skin, the sensation of being delivered/released replaces the sensation of immobilization. From the grimace as sensation returns to my extremities, to the great sigh of relief, to the smile that follows—deliverance comes in many forms! My partner and I may admire together the esoteric details—the marks that often indicate the ferocity of the submissive. We don't worry about them; they will disappear by themselves in a few minutes or a few hours. A massage can aid in regaining normal circulation.

"There you are," I say. "It is over." Everything went smoothly, and we are both exhausted and still highly excited at the same time. It is a time for pure intimacy, like the calm after the storm. A release from all suffering involves three words: tenderness, relaxation, silence.

I reassure myself that my love is doing well. We sit up a little to drink together. I gather the ropes while she looks at the drawings.... It is time to thank each other, to confide in one another, to share some light laughter. We benefit from massaging spots that are still sore on each other, using fine oils or lotions.

Let's take the time to come back to Earth, to utter our first reviews.

What's important for me is to thank my love for experiencing these moments with me, these tingles of pleasures, and (if it is the case) for the pretty drawings I've made with Chinese ink.

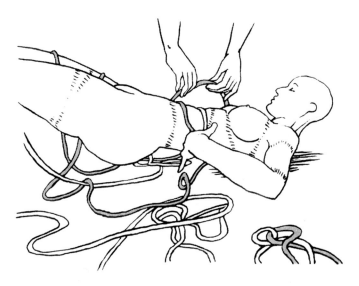

Allow freeing your partner to feel as sensuous as binding her.

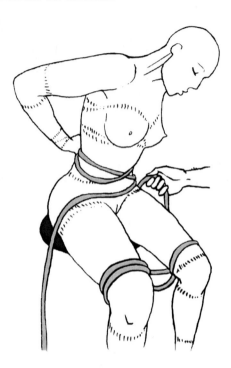

**Assure your partner—and yourself—that any marks
left over from play will be gone shortly.**

◉ **Memories, Memories** The realization that the perfect bondage is a work of art, as pleasing in gestures as it is in
spectacle, which you—the one doing the tying—have created.
But what is left of all this when it is time to untie the knots
and free your submissive? The memories...but the kind of
memories that you can't share with even your partner. Because
the role of each participant is so different from the other, your
experiences—and your memories—will also be different.

Why not savor memories of these moments? A photo representing your work (of art) may be a good souvenir for both of you. Glue it into your personal diary, away from wandering eyes. For me, I never post anything online (Big Brother is watching). I say a little more perversity could do us all some good: I am thinking of using some photos (or a film) of this session for the next one, to make my next playmate sing out or offer more of herself....

The moment can last.

As for drawings, you will need to demonstrate some speed as well as dexterity as the model will rarely last more than four or five minutes in the position into which you have stretched her. Still, the value of an original drawing done "on the spot," even if not very detailed, adds to the jubilation of our little game....

Below, a pretty "X" describes for us her meeting with Frank. She is fully submissive to him. He begins undressing her and then moves on to serious things. And he has more than one trick in his bag.

> "It is a scarf, and he blindfolds my eyes. I let him slide me onto the bed. I am laid out at present, my eyes covered and my hands over my breasts. He has something else in his briefcase, but this time I don't get to see anything more. I feel him tying my wrist; he spreads my arms away from my body to tie them at each side of the bed, as to a cross. The silence is almost sacred. I let myself go, knowing that after this point I cannot defend myself.
>
> "That is just what I am looking for: Choice taken away from me, the ability to get away depends on

him alone. He removes my bra. If I were to make a move to stop him, it would be of no use for I am well tied down.

"Now he is caressing the length of my body, lingering on my breasts. His mouth is everywhere, softly, and I let myself enjoy it...not only do I enjoy it, but I enjoy the anticipation of what comes next. I want it so bad that it scares me.

"I hear him get something. He ties my legs to either side of the bed; thus splayed open I know that I am completely at his mercy. There is no question of escape. Once again he takes his time caressing me and mouthing me with infinite delicacy. I feel bad that I am exposed in nudity; happily, I don't have to look at myself...his lips trace up my legs, arriving sweetly uninterrupted at my sex. The man kisses my lower cleft and tongues his way around inside me. At first it was too much, and I tried to pull my legs together. But very quickly this feeling changed to a strong desire. He intentionally draws it out. Finally, his mouth comes to rest covering my sex. I feel his tongue wiggling, and it gently explores my depth as my heart leaps. I know he will find my clitoris after driving me mad with anticipation. He acts like a master who knows all there is to know about women. I want to suck him, but my sense of modesty gets in the way. His tongue flicks on my clitoris, and his soft breath there makes me tremble...."

Ch 6. Scenarios

The imagination is without limits. Don't you agree?

The bedroom is essentially the preferred setting for all sorts of frolicking. Or, if one can find the right time and company, there are other places for being naughty.

The kitchen and the laundry room take on a new charm when one puts a woman on top of the washer for the spin cycle.... The garage smells better, of liquids and lubricants hidden among the tools that can be used for erotica—only with a condom, obviously! And the attic! The dust is dreamy. You can try the cupboard, a storage bin, the boss's office, the dentist and his most important furnishing, the chair!

Add to this a few clever games like:

- escape artist
- come at the same time
- tickle torture: a must! (using fingers, a feather, a feather-duster, a paintbrush, etc.)
- submissive furniture: tied in poses like chair, coat rack, etc.
- take advantage of the situation to—only with permission—shave the head of the poor maid, or her privates, or even apply a few lashes with the whip to satisfy the lion tamer in you!

☞ just as nice and much softer, try every sort of dessert top-
  ping—natural or sugary—or champagne for toasting to the
  experience when you have completed the session

Here are a few thoughts to keep in mind:

☞ Don't forget that a submissive in good condition should
  and must take orders without flinching, or else there will
  be punishment!
☞ Take time to absorb the simply magnificent: What could
  be more exciting than laying out a beautiful body, exqui-
  sitely bound, on an exotic fur blanket?
☞ Making love uninhibitedly is a fine idea; making love with
  restraints is, too.

You will find some suggestions for scenarios and fantasies
to create in the following passages. The drawings should give
you some good ideas, too. Understand that the list is limited
but your imagination is not, and your own fantasies will provide you with the most rewarding experiences!

THE PROCRASTINATOR

"You aren't just one or two…you are three minutes
late! Thanks to you, we are missing the beginning
of the play **The Vagina Monologues**! Thanks a
lot! So, for those three minutes, I will treat you to
another game. It is called 'the anus monologue'!
And soon you will be starring in it. No chance you
will miss the beginning of this one! Ha! Ha! Ha!"

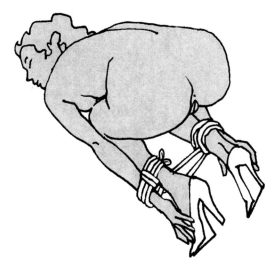

**With such a sweet package at your feet,
you're bound to enjoy yourself.**

SAUSAGED

"My but you are beautiful strapped tight, my sweet Kaori! You are the most exciting woman my hands have ever been on! What patience! What resistance to pain! You blow my mind! I'm going to lay you on the bed and begin the exploration of your body. My fingers can't wait to trace lines on your skin; my tongue quivers with longing. I'm going to take an hour to look at every inch of you...above and below...between...around...inside! You are so beautiful. It's going to be ecstasy!"

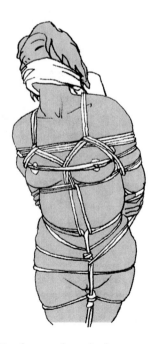

**Bondage can leave both master
and submissive aching for more.**

THE SERVANT

"I'm to be punished. My master didn't care for the careless smudges I left on the crystal. I did my best to polish them, but here I am anyway tied to this wretched iron bed and on this miserable old mattress. What a nightmare! The worst is when he calmly tends to my ass…oh! It is so humiliating to be on exhibit in front of my master and his friends…."

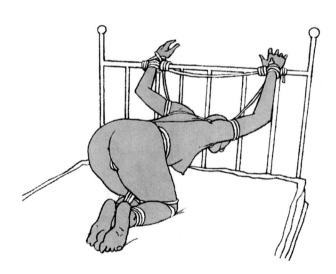

**With your submissive bound before you,
your mind swims with possibilities….**

"PUBIC" CHAIR

"This guy is nuts! I'm really scared. How did I get talked into coming here? I know what it is...I was duped! This character...you say, he acted like an artist or a painter...more like a voyeur and a pervert! I never should have agreed to this! I'm such a sap. And my arms are starting to hurt...I'm too arched; I'm gonna feel it tomorrow! And him, he'll use it as an excuse to run around getting laid...you can bet he won't be making sketches! He'll rut!

"I can sense, he approaches.... If he ever touches me! What a horror...ohhh... he is so close; he is caressing my slit.... Get your dirty hands off me...he stops...wait!... Ohhh...do it again...I want more...come and take me... come on...I want it!"

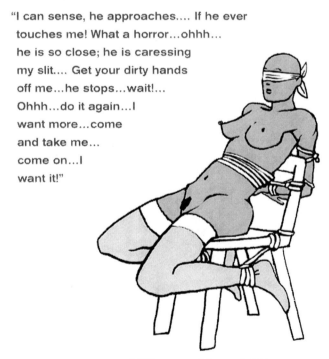

A little sense of danger heightens our feelings of anticipation.

ON YOUR KNEES!

"Martine made a bore of herself at our last dinner with
the Durands. She said
more than five sentences
over the course of the
evening—more than
we had agreed to ear-
lier. Therefore, she
must be punished:
on her knees in the
armchair, her fig
exposed and her
gaze directed far
above the imple-
ment with which
I will punish her
rump: champagne,
semen, whipped
cream, a prod...."

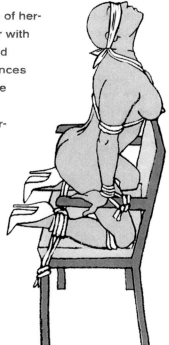

**The addition of the blindfold
makes my partner quiver.**

SLAVE

"On this our anniversary, Max gave me a strange
gift: A playmate that says, 'Yes'—a living doll,
a man!

"All right, babe! To start with, see to my holes.
Admire them, feel them...oh! I have to tinkle! A
golden shower! Naturally, it is spring! A storm
shower."

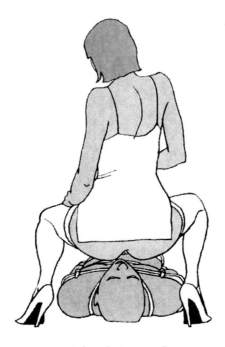

Aah, to be in control!

COFFEE TABLE

"Daphne just arrived. I have all I need to forgive her for her last caprice at dance class: That goose dared to dance with every other partner in the class except me! She thinks she is better than me! Only by smoothing over some of her rough patches can I appease my thirst for vengeance. Once I get her tied down, I'll spread her open and pierce, explore, excited, but I will only bring her to the brink of orgasm, nothing more."

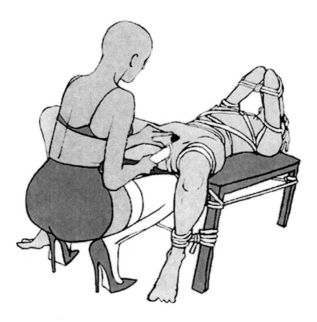

Oh, the fun that adding props can bring.

SING OUT

"It has been a half hour since Lea, my singing
coach, started diddling my organ with the end of
her riding crop. I have sung every song I know as
best as I can, but she is never satis-
fied! I can't take any more. I never
can hit those high notes!...It's
impossible! And she knows
it, that bitch! Ouch, another
slap!...Oh! That burns...
it hurts...stop...ouch!...
Aaaah...."

**The sting of my dominance will
turn sweet for my partner.**

Conclusion

The day when I discovered that binding someone can open doors to spiritual and sensual spaces in another dimension, I began an unending journey. Through this book, I hope I've convinced you to give it a chance, too!

And there is still one more thing: The best way to appreciate the sensation of being held in ropes is to take a leap and allow yourself to be tied…be DAREing! DARE to be bound. Feel the caress of rope on your skin and the indescribable pressure created by the ropes squeezing your mounds together. Allow yourself to be corseted, to be scolded, to be splayed open and at the mercy of madam's wishes…taste the timeless experience of being wrapped in heavy Oriental fabrics!

Then, and only then, can you test the dangerous currents of the master's role!

Remember: The master is no better than the slave he was.…

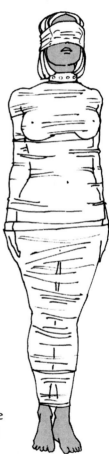

The beauty—and anticipation—of the bound body.

Glossary of Bondage

It is hard enough to speak when one is gagged—even harder in Japanese. Nevertheless, here are some elements of vocabulary that belong to Shibari. A good number of expressions used in this manual do not translate neatly (into English). Regardless, it is preferred—and infinitely more high-class—to use the Japanese terms to discuss and describe the practices we have come to know here. The vocabulary that follows also includes the current terminology of the scene—clothing, action verbs—and certain bondage poses found in this guide. I thank my friend Yoko for sharing some of her secrets—her linguistic secrets—with us.

Agura: Crossed legs (Lotus)
Ashitote musubi: Hands and feet tied
Asanawa: Linen rope
Dorei: Slave
Gyaku-ebi: The inverted prawn
Kaikyaku kani: Crab (with legs spread open)
Karada: Harness that envelopes the body
Kikkou: Tortoise shell—diamond—harness for the upper body (bust)
Kinbaku: The art of tying
Mae okurimono: Exposed from the front
Makurae: Erotic Japanese print
Mune nawa: Tying the breasts
Musubime: Knot

Nawashi: Artist of rope
Sakuranbo: Genital restriction (squeezed tight)
Sensei: Master
Shibari: Tying
Shinju: The Pearls—bondage of the breasts
Tsuri-zeme: Torture of suspension
Unsui: Student
Ushiro okurimono: Exposed from behind
Yukata: Kimono of cotton

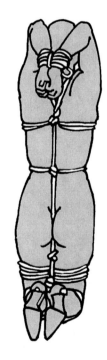

**There are so many ways
to bind and explore.**

Bibliography

Books

Djian, Philippe. *Vers chez les blancs* (Lines of White). Coll. Folio, Gallimard, 2000.

Ficelle, Tonton, illustrator. *Contraintes*. Presented by Jean-Claude Baboulin and Annabel Faust. Paris: Editions Alixe, 1998.

Love, Brenda B. *Dictionnaire des fantasmes, perversions, et pratiques de l'amour* (Dictionary of Fantasies, Perversions, and Love Practices). Paris: Editions Blanche, 2000.

Resources

Reference Books
Wiseman, Jay. *Erotic Bondage Handbook*. Greenery Press, 2000.

Photograph Books
Bondage: Laura Manson Stansfield Photocollection, Goliath, 2005.
Castro, Rick. *13 Years of Bondage: The Photography of Rick Castro.*
    Fluxion, 2004.
Lee, Edward, coll. *Bondage: Erotic Art of Rope*. Extrahot, Mixofpix,
    2004.
Speliotis, Steven. *Asia Bondage.* Goliath, 2003.
Any works by Nobuyoshi, which are odes to the virtue of bondage.

Illustrated Books/Cartoons
Axterdam. *Carnets d'un obsédé* (An Obsessed Person's Notebook).
    La Musardine, 2003.
Baldazzini, Roberto, and Franco Saudelli. *Bizarreries.* Glittering
    Images, 2002.
Kondom. *Bondage Fairies.* Eros Comix, 2001.
Saudelli, Franco. *The Bondage Clinic and Foot Fantasies.* Glittering
    Images, 1992.
Saudelli, Franco. *Franco Bondage Archive, #1: Tied and Tickled.* Glit-
    tering Images, 1998.
Saudelli, Franco. *Franco Bondage Archive, #2: Chair Ties.* Glittering
    Images, 1998.

Saudelli, Franco. *The Bondage Clinic and the Fetishistic Gang.* Glittering Images, 2001.

Saudelli, Franco. *Barefoot and Bondage Photo Fantasies.* Glittering Images, 2003.

Willie, John. *Sweet Gwendoline.* Belier Press, 1995.

Websites
www.altsex.org/bdsm
www.tieguyuk.com
www.tes.org

Films
Bondage Classic 1, by Irving Klaw.
Bondage Classic 2, by Irving Klaw.
Betty Page, Bondage Queen, by Irving Klaw.
The Embryo Hunts in Secret, directed by Wakamatsu Koji, 1966.
Gwendoline, directed by Just Jaeckin, 1984.
The Nightcomers, directed by Michaël Winner, 1972.
Nikutai No Mon (Gate of Flesh), directed by Seijun Suzuki, 1964.

Sex Toy Retailers
Adam and Eve, www.adameve.com
Eve's Garden, www.evesgarden.com
Good Vibrations, www.goodvibes.com
Toys in Babeland, www.babeland.com

CPSIA information can be obtained at www.ICGtesting.com
Printed in the USA
LVOW07s1457231015

459499LV00017B/333/P